A Sight to Behold

Copyright 2011 Greta Bryan
All rights reserved.

ISBN-10: 1460948777
EAN-13: 9781460948774

A Sight to Behold

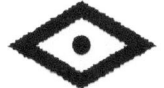

Greta Bryan

Dedicated to

My husband, Albert H. (Hal) Bryan, MD,
who brought sight to many

and

Lowell Gess, MD,
who provided the first opportunity

THE VISION

Freetown, Sierra Leone, West Africa

"It was 1976 and I was on my way to do eye surgery upcountry at the Lunsar Eye Hospital. My road circled Mount Leicester. On that day, it was clear. As I moved to the open side of the road, I could see the bustling city lying at my feet with traffic movement resembling little ants. During the dry season, the backdrop is brown, but with the rains, greenery springs up everywhere. After viewing the breathtaking scene for a period, I was suddenly struck with the realization that there were a million people at my feet. Along with the more than ten million people of West Africa, they needed modern eye care. In that moment I felt a Christian compassion that prompted a resolve to continue a yearly volunteer eye ministry to Sierra Leone for as long as the Lord would lend me breath."

Lowell Gess, MD
MINE EYES HAVE SEEN THE GLORY

Table of Contents

Prologue xi
In the Beginning. 1
A Sight to Behold 9
Fearing the Fall. 13
On an Easter Morning in Sierra Leone 29
The Way It Was and Still Is 33
Ghana Diary. 43
Haiti 55
Eyes on the Philippines 69
Doctor, Heal Thyself 71
Creatures of the Night. 81
Rockin' and Rollin' 83
And finally.... 93
The Clinics 97
Destinations. 99
Definitions 101

Prologue

In 1982, my husband, Dr. Hal Bryan, in private practice for eleven years, was examining his life and asking, "Is this it...is this all there is? I'm a successful ophthalmologist, but emotionally, something is missing."

Three events changed his life.

First: In a sermon, Reverend Dan Smith, the pastor in our Methodist church, told this story: A young man finished his college education and was offered a high-paying job as an engineer in a well-established firm, but turned it down; instead, he decided to use his skills in a Third World country. The CEO questioned his decision, saying, "Why are you throwing all that you've worked for in that environment? Is it the money? Can we offer you a bigger salary?"

And the young man said, "Oh, it's not the salary. It's the job that is not big enough."

Dr. Bryan mused about that: he was successful, the salary was big enough, but somehow in his heart the job was not big enough, not satisfying.

Second: Dr. Vic Pentz, Presbyterian minister, spoke at our daughter's high school graduation and challenged the students to get a degree attached to a usable skill that can be carried to a Third World country and used to ease the need.

Third: The next day after graduation, Dr. Lowell Gess's letter arrived, requesting donations to build a clinic in Sierra Leone, West Africa, and donations of time to serve in the clinic. Dr. Bryan answered both calls.

Dr. Bryan carried on his mission work for fifteen years, giving sight to hundreds of people, but the patients gave us much more; they allowed us to see what is truly important in life.

In the Beginning
1984

In May of 1984, my husband and I returned home from a unique volunteer effort, which culminated in Sierra Leone, a small country in western Africa, 7,500 miles away from Washington State. Dr. Lowell Gess, a Minnesota ophthalmologist who has spent years in African medical mission work, was able to obtain donations from ophthalmologists and other donors in the states and carpenter hours from South Dakota volunteers to build the Kissy Eye Clinic, located in a Methodist church compound in the small town of Kissy Mess-Mess (appropriately named, I might add) outside of Freetown, the capital.

Considering there were only two permanent ophthalmologists in the entire country, you can imagine the need. We prepared for the trip for over a year since Dr. Bryan was responsible for not only financing the trip but for collecting medical supplies from various generous drug companies around the country. For six weeks prior to our departure, our basement resembled fertile ground for a drug bust. Our hometown church, Wesley Methodist, donated $6,000 toward equipment. By the time we were finally ready to haul ourselves to the Seattle airport on April 4, we tallied arm-wrenching carry-ons plus five hundred pounds of supplies with enough leftover room for a camera, a few changes of clothes, cereal for Hal, and toilet paper—all stashed into seven carefully weighed and measured cardboard apple boxes, stacked in twos and secured by donated custom-made straps.

Our greatest stress during the planning months was caused by the rumor that medical supplies were often confiscated by custom officials at the Monrovian airport in Liberia, our first stop. Since we had to stay there overnight before flying on to Sierra Leone, we had visions of losing everything and being forced to abruptly end our mission. Our travel agent and I contacted our congressman, who made the right phone calls and, believe it or not, the system worked. A young, congenial African man, holding a piece of paper with our names on it, was waiting for us when our plane landed in Liberia, then whisked us through customs, hauled our boxes to a nearby hotel, and even came back the next day to make sure we were on our way.

Welcome to Africa.

A short plane ride and a river ferry separated us from Liberia and our destination, Freetown, an environment teeming with 400,000 people, many of them bare-breasted, sarong-skirted women with baskets and barrels of produce piled high with more weight than any two of us could carry, propped in perfect balance on top of their heads. They often had babies secured to their backs and one on the way bulging from the front.

We learned early on that cleanliness registered next to nothing. We witnessed culture shock of the first order, driving down the narrow streets of Freetown for the first time midst throngs of people and open sewers running down either side of the street. The water was the result of, and used for, an assortment of daily functions.

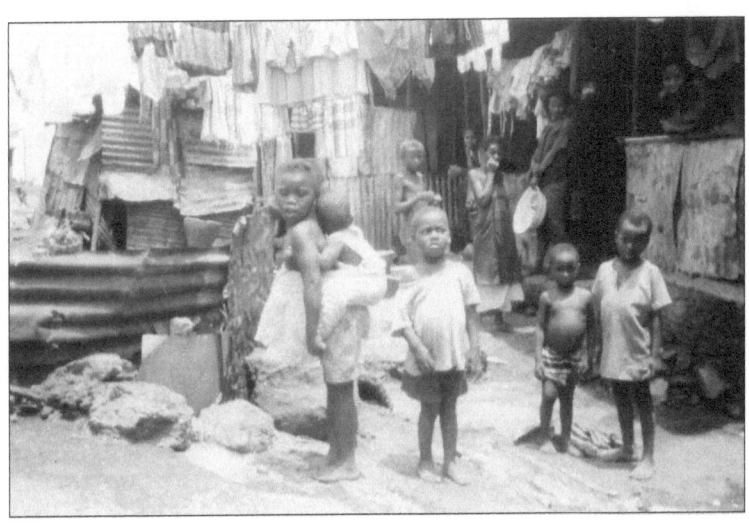

It's a tough life for kids

The craziness of the streets caused us to visit a landmark we'd not planned...the police station; the day was Sierra Leone's version of our Fourth of July (April 19). We were slowly edging down a side street when two policemen roared up alongside. Thinking we were going too slowly, we motioned them to go around us. Wrong. They wanted words with us.

Charge: driving the wrong way on a one-way street **past** the police station. Tense moments followed. Why were we in the country? How long? Didn't we **know** about one-way streets? Long pauses. Then we uttered the magic words: Dr. Gess and the Kissy Eye Clinic. Broad smiles quickly replaced intimidating questioning. Verdict: a warning from them and a promise from us for new eye glasses at the clinic. (You scratch my back...I'll scratch yours.)

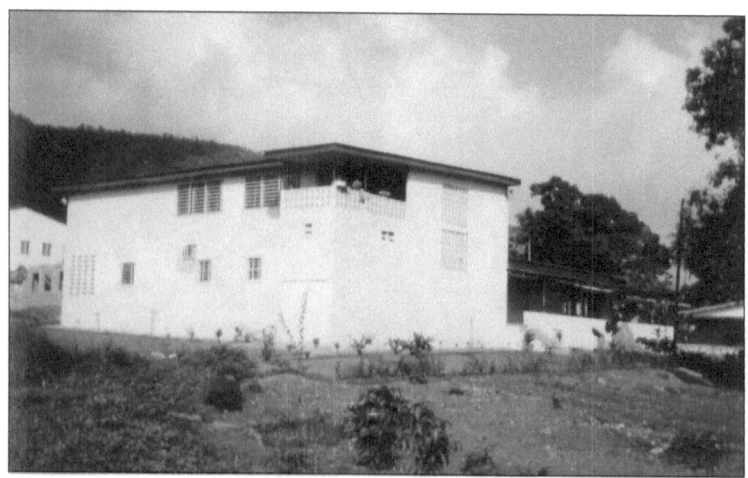

Kissy Eye Clinic

The Kissy Eye Clinic, only one of several buildings within the walled Methodist Mission compound, stood as the newest, however. A sweep through the front door took us into the waiting room, complete with benches, an optical shop, and a bathroom. On down the corridor, we went into a small examining room, then straight back to two recovery rooms, a laundry room, and the operating theatre. Meanwhile, going outside and up a flight of stairs brought us to our living quarters.

The clinic and surrounding grounds were guarded at night by Joseph. Supposedly. More often than not, he could be caught sleeping on the front porch by ten o' clock unless we stuffed him with a peanut-butter sandwich. The only thing he loved more than peanut butter was his torch (flashlight) which he used with abandonment.

The gifts of growing mango and banana trees alongside the clinic did not escape our eyes, nor did the spectacular termite hills reaching to the roofline of the clinic! We learned the queen sits royally deep in the well of the hill, eating and producing, while the workers spend their entire lives feeding her, undoubtedly dragging the food from the footings of the clinic!

Forty to sixty patients, five to eleven surgeries per day, made only a crease in the problem. Dense cataracts, lost or nearly lost eyes due to glaucoma or measles. The patience and courage of these patients will not be forgotten;

they started lining up outside the clinic at 5:00 a.m. and waited. Relatives helped struggling blind relatives, mothers nursed their babies, and old men dozed. Dr. Bryan was gratefully aided by John, a permanent staff scrub nurse, Leticia, an ophthalmic nurse trained in London, and Jonathon, the maintenance man, scrubber of floors, laundry man, and general gofer.

The babies, their brown faces topped with black brillo-like pads, captured our hearts. The mothers came to the compound's maternity ward to deliver and eat a hot meal ($5 US), sometimes leaving in the dead of night **without** the baby.

As we walked into Freetown's Musselman Memorial Church on our first Sunday in Africa, the congregation was singing...and when Africans sing, they open their mouths wide and let it all roll out in three-part harmony! The women sat on the left side, men on the right; we slipped in and sat together in the back but were quickly invited up front. Thankfully. We were rewarded with the full tilt of their singing **and** it was cooler. The preacher introduced us:

"Who know Dr. Gess?"

"You know...eye...eye."

Hands went up.

"Praise de Lor."

"Now here doctor here to take care of eye. Praise de Lor. Dr Gess leave...Dr. Boelke come...now Dr. Boelke leave and Dr. Bryan come. Praise de Lor. For 25 cents... for 10 cents...go in...fix eye...come back. Praise de Lor."

We sat down, duly introduced.

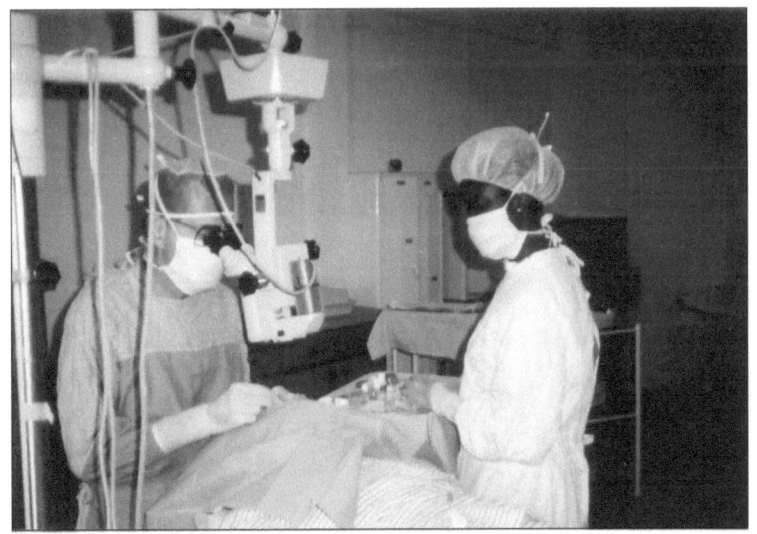

Dr. Bryan and scrub nurse Leticia

Postscript:

A Lebanese businessman and his extended and extensive family, patients as well as significant financial benefactors of the Kissy Clinic, became our friends. They invited us into their homes, fed us, drove us on outings, held long conversations with us, discussed their Islamic faith, and listened attentively as we shared our Christian faith. On our first trip to Sierra Leone, we had to fly first to Monrovia, Liberia, as well as return there en route to the U.S. They arranged to have one of their relatives meet us at the Monrovian airport to ensure our safety, then again fed us and waited until we were safely on the plane heading home.

We remain grateful to them.

A Sight to Behold

Under the surgical drape, only his quiet left eye was revealed. A dense cataract had kept him blind for twenty years. Now it appeared as a white opaque marble held stationary by local anesthesia. Though he didn't show any emotion, Amandu was scared, fearing what many African patients fear—that the doctor was going to remove his eye, wash it off, and put it back in.

But for now, Amandu Bangura appeared asleep, not from general anesthesia but from weariness, no doubt aided by the comfort of a bed in the cool operating room. After all, he and his nephew had walked ten kilometers to get to the Kissy Eye Clinic, a Mecca for eye care, sorely needed in this African country of Sierra Leone. News of the American surgical team's arrival traveled quickly.

His above-average height allowed me to remember seeing Amandu that morning. He joined hundreds of

African patients, who, like ants racing in and out of their hills in search of food for their queen, streamed in from the city streets and villages, down dusty paths, their thongs and bare feet pushing clouds of red dirt off their heels, focusing their energies on getting to the clinic. The tall white doctor was their hope for sight.

Amandu was among the first to arrive, long before the sun had risen to meet the day, clutching the arm of his nephew, Foday, a rail-thin youngster, ten or twelve years old. It's hard to determine age in Africa, where one often doesn't enjoy two meals in one day.

Though Foday's ragged Dallas Cowboys T-shirt hung limply off lean shoulders, Amandu's dress code was more formal: a long-sleeved, ankle-length, pale blue cotton tunic, once enhanced, now frayed by darker embroidery at the collarless neck and sleeve hems. On closer inspection, what had appeared to be a tie-dye project were actually splotchy memories of food and body functions. Perched on his white natural Afro and adding another four inches to his reedy frame was a well-coiled faded turban.

After many hours of quiet waiting, he was directed to the operating table. Now the surgeon's hands rested on his forehead, poised for the first incision. The sterile drape moved in rhythm to his mouth breathing, forcing it to rise and fall around his mouth and nose. The drape was a blessing. His breath, unfiltered, would stop a train.

Cleaning his face prior to surgery introduced me to each line etched in his narrow, sunken face; small unseeing eyes hunkered under bushy brows, the white stubble on his upper lip and chin, and his colorless cracked lips hovering over the only tooth in his head.

His feet fascinated me; two nails missing, his soles no stranger to the miles of ground he'd covered during his eighty-two years. The gnarled arthritic knuckles of his hand, which grasped the head of his walking stick that morning, now rested quietly at his side.

Yes, for now he was at peace, perhaps even dreaming of a new tomorrow.

Postscript:
When his patch was taken off the next morning, and he was able to see, he turned first to Dr. Bryan and asked, "What you **do**?" Then he turned to Foday and berated him for not taking better care of him!

Fearing the Fall
Sierra Leone, West Africa

" Sierra Leone is in the great crisis in history. This once beautiful and cultural jewel of West Africa is now in the throes of an internal war. The rebels known as the Revolutionary United Front under Foday Sankow are step by step taking over rural Sierra Leone as Charles Taylor did in Liberia five years ago. They move from place to place at will, killing especially village leaders and then burning their homes. By intimidation, they force teenagers to join their ranks who then are caught up in the ritual of killing and destroying. They keep themselves supplied by looting.

It is never known how often their AK47s are real and functional.

All hospitals and health centers up country have been closed with all its equipment and large supply of medicines looted by the rebels; only the Kissy UMC Eye Hospital is in operation in Freetown."

In a letter from Dr. Lowell Gess, 1995

I wonder how many Americans are losing sleep over the news from Sierra Leone, West Africa. My husband and I are.

The Kissy Eye Clinic is located in the district of Kissy, Sierra Leone, on narrow, abused, drive-at-your-own risk road from Freetown, the capital. The clinic celebrated completion in 1984, thanks to Dr. Lowell Gess, Minnesota ophthalmologist and African missionary, and legends of volunteers. Since then thousands of Africans have stumbled into the clinic, blinded by cataracts, and walked away with their sight. We have been part of that miracle of medicine.

And now? Civil war has produced uniformed and armed bands who have robbed, looted, raped, and killed without conscience. The government hospital and the Kissy Eye Clinic were in their direct path of destruction.

"Augustine, the clinic's optician, was stopped last week by an 11-year-old with an AK47, demanding sweets. Fortunately, for Augustine, an argument erupted a few feet

away. The young boy moved over and executed one of them. People are afraid to appear on the streets during the day and spend sleepless nights awaiting the invasion of their homes. Many of the staff have gone three or four days without food. Their greatest fear is being summarily and randomly executed. Some are able to flee to remote places up-country while others have slipped across borders to neighboring countries."

In a letter from Dr. Gess. February 1999

I often awaken in the early morning and wonder about the fate of our young and old friends and patients whose stories have silenced audiences in our Washington hometown. And then I remember the first month we spent in Kissy. April 1984.

Smell is what's missing in the telling. Thinking of a country-sized, ripe compost helps in describing our introduction to Freetown's overpopulated, never-sleeping streets. Our sheltered, naïve American eyes stared in disbelief at the squalid neighborhood shacks, the desperate, dirty, ragged street vendors hawking their livelihoods, brazen unrestrained goats, mangy dogs, and naked kids darting in and out of traffic, leading with distended bellies and herniated navels. All of this, breeding and boiling under the relentless noonday sun, was a stark contrast to the air-conditioned Mercedes Benz-carpooling government officials honking through intersections. Their biggest challenge was dodging tire-sized potholes, which sat neglected on streets flanked by gutters. These public cesspools were filled to street level with swampy water of questionable origins and used in more ways than we wanted to think about. The hairs in my nose burned.

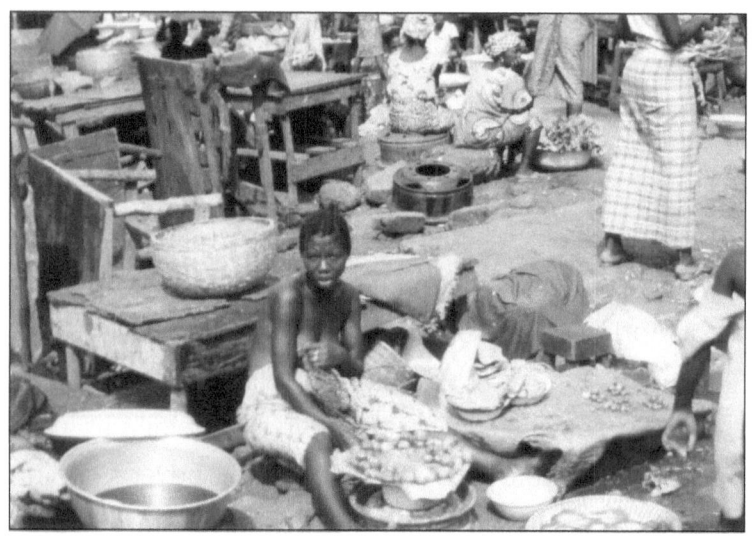

A woman trader on the streets of Freetown

My dry mouth hung open as I watched from our crowded Toyota the overburdened, underappreciated women, straight sweaty backs, necks wide, heavy containers of palm oil or baskets of seasonal fruits and vegetables balanced on their braided heads. They strode rhythmically, stretching the seams of their ankle length sarongs tied at waists, full dark heavy breasts swinging freely. All seemingly unnoticed. Many of the women sat at the side of the road straddling their produce and handcrafts, swatting flies from the fresh fish, and minding their babies, who only had to whimper to be rewarded with a leisurely pull at a familiar, engorged breast.

Catching our eye as we waited, wedged in a predictable traffic jam, was a tall, pathetic-looking adolescent. His chest was sunken, his young black eyes registered unbearable pain, and his left foot seeped pus from a swollen open wound. The color of our skin suggested help. After lifting his foot for our inspection, he dropped his ragged pants and without hesitation or embarrassment, showed us his penis. That is, what was left of it. It was chopped off to within an inch. We didn't ask how or why. Instead, we pleaded with him to come to the clinic to get a shot of penicillin. Although he smiled a knowing sad smile, and gave us a positive nod to assure us he understood, he never showed up.

Why didn't we just pack him into the car and take him to the clinic? I don't know. The memory of his ravaged body still haunts me.

At every corner, we witnessed the hardships of congenital birth defects, of useless arms and legs hanging and turning at impossible angles. Equally dramatic were the albinos. The first time I met Mama Sesay, she was sitting on a flat rock at the edge of the clinic's walled compound. Her pendulous breasts hung bare while a tie-dyed scarf circled the crown of her balding head. A faded floral wraparound skirt was drawn up between her legs like a cellist in an orchestra. She sat stirring rice. Her nudity was not what I noticed first, but rather her pale, pinkish, watery eyes and blotched, unpigmented skin. Her stretched and mottled leathery breasts rested like worn shoe soles on her bloated belly. Checking **me** out was an assortment of young women, a few pregnant, some nursing, others fussing with their hair.

Unsupervised children raced about, scratching, picking their noses and other body parts, while chewing on whatever they could find. All were related to Mama in some way. Behind the fire pit was her shack, which leaned gratefully against the head-high compound wall. Considering there was no door on the shack, it was easy to take a quick inventory and see the entire six-foot square of tin and other street-finds welded together to give it hope. The glance also revealed one iron bed with a thin sheetless mattress, one small table under a hole in the wall pretending to be a window, woven grass mats, a large blackened pot, and little else. Mama noticed my inquiring look, smiled her toothless smile, and assured me that she always had first dibs on the one bed. The shack's other occupants varied from night to night.

No room for sissies here.

"A ploy often used is to come to a home and offer protection if the people would agree to care for them, which they did. When ready to move on, certain people in the home were ordered to pick up slips of paper with instructions written on them. The notes offered choices hard to imagine: 'cut off right hand' or 'cut off left arm' or 'kill this one' or 'let this one go,' 'cut off right ear' or 'put out left eye'. There are 2000 amputees in Freetown. It is estimated that only 20 to 25 percent of those suffering atrocities are able to seek help before they die of complications. The houses and business apartments along Kissy Road stand naked, burned out walls…"
In a letter from Dr. Gess, June 1998

I remember the large angry pimple festering in the middle of Joseph's forehead when he showed up at the clinic on our first night in Kissy in 1984. Then I noticed the white corneal scars on both eyes, a memory of childhood measles. Ten years old. His father was dead, and his mother lived up-country with his siblings, which left Joseph to shift his meager possessions in and out of the shacks of friends or an available uncle. His exposed ribs spoke of meals missed, but his passion was not for a full belly but rather for a bike and schooling. The chance of owning a bike was slim to none, but we stepped up to make his second dream come true. But not without a few setbacks.

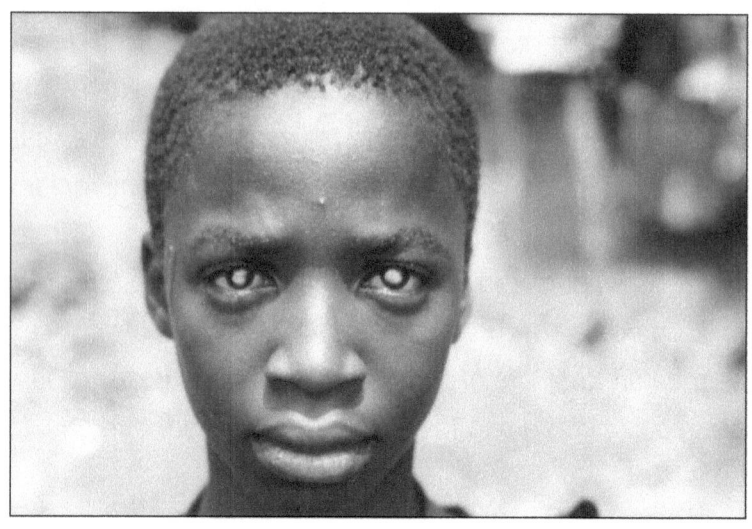

Joseph with corneal scars due to measles

"Greta…you sent my fee through my head teacher, Teacher Tombo. The last time you sent dollars for my school purpose in care of Teacher to give to me for school purpose but the teacher who I can call dishonest and greedy man hold it for himself. Please Greta I want you to assist so that I can go back to school and educated and be a good man in future. I hope my letter will you favorable consider."
Joseph's letter, 1989

"Early this month Dr. Bryan learned that a corneal transplant by another visiting U.S. ophthalmologist restored full vision in Joseph's left eye. Now happiness has turned to tragedy. Today we learned he has fallen victim to violence, resulting in the loss of that prized eye."
             Journal, 1993

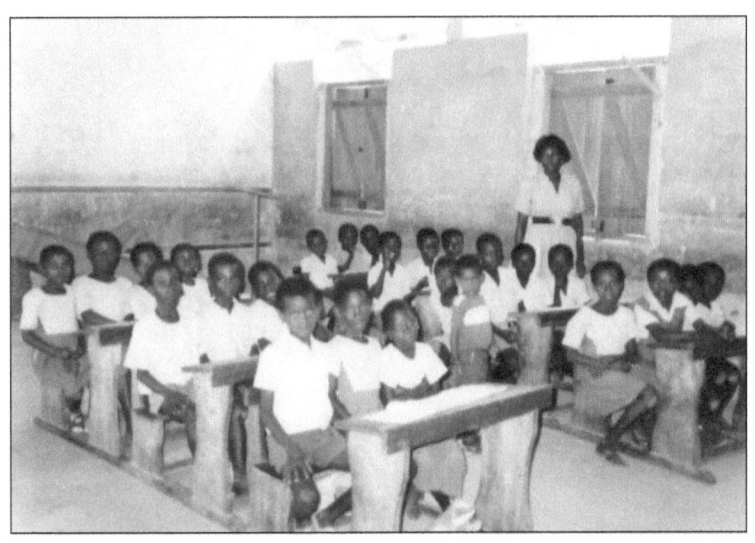

Kids in a crowded classroom

I fear for Foday, a tall, strapping kid, later a handsome young man with fire and determination in his soul to get educated and better his life. I wonder where and how he is. We met Foday on our first journey to Sierra Leone in 1984. Shannon, our daughter, a senior in high school, went with us for the first two weeks and helped in the clinic. She and Foday became friends. We funded his education and now pray for him.

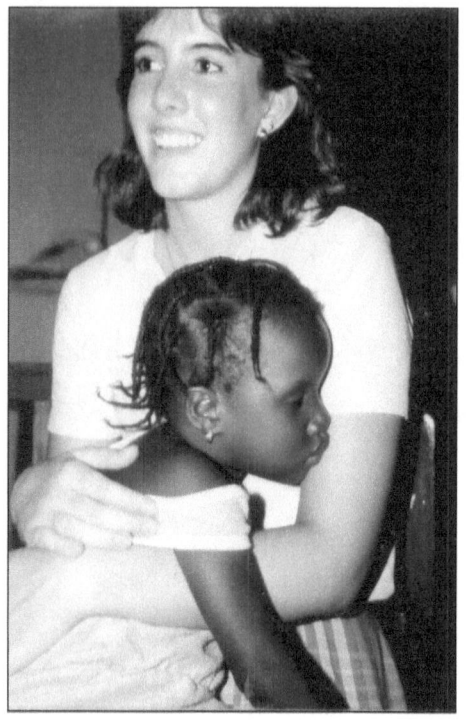

Daughter Shannon and a tired little girl

"Greta, this revolution in Sierra Leone has caused a lot of destruction in my life and the country. It is almost three months since the military take over the country. There is no work, no school and no other business going on in the country. Everything has gone to standstill. There is continuous harassment of people, looting of properties, raping of

woman and killing people. Then the students decided to make a peaceful demonstration to say no to the military junta and back to the democratically elected government but they turn against us and started arresting the students. Up to the time I was leaving Freetown, all students were in hiding because if a student is caught, they will beat him mercilessly and then take him to the central prison. This threat force me to leave the country. I don't know when I will write to you again. God bless you all."

Last letter from Foday, August 26, 1997

And the others?

Is Peter able to cope?

"I cry all night, my wife, she cry. I only thirty years and have to know if I going blind. If I blind I keel myself. I am a teacher. My heart it is ha-vee. I must know my fault." Peter was told that macular degeneration does not result in total blindness; he would still have his side vision. But is he able to cope?

We later learned that teachers go regularly on strike. They don't get paid for months. I asked Sully, a young African friend, if the teachers demonstrated. He said they'd probably be shot if they did. Where is rail-thin Jonathan, a faithful employee since opening day of the clinic? Because he sent most of his meager wages to his family up-country, he had to share a corner of a communal shack alongside thirteen others. He maneuvered a scrub mop and short-handled broom around the clinic floor, challenging the tracks of red dirt as well as taking care of the laundry. His wide infectious grin never registered a complaint. He, like the rest of the staff at the clinic, felt the good fortune of having a job.

Is Andrew still alive? We found eight-year-old Andrew crying quietly outside the clinic the first week. He had walked his blind sister to surgery and was now waiting for her. When questioned, he reluctantly showed us a severe scalding covering most of his back! He was immediately taken care of and for the next three weeks continued to come by daily for clean dressing and, even more important to him, peanut butter sandwiches.

Did the wrinkled, wailing baby, born to a terrified fourteen-year-old survive? In the cool of early morning, serenaded by the aggravating but dependable rooster and Muslims chanting their morning prayers, I slipped into the adjacent building, which housed the busy maternity ward. I watched in awe as the mini, matted head of the baby crowned. The tired midwife held the baby girl up and announced to the empty room, in big tones, "Her name be Greta!" Mama didn't have the strength to argue. Later that night, Mama disappeared into the darkness of the city. Without Baby Greta. Do you suppose she thought I would take care of my namesake? I wonder.

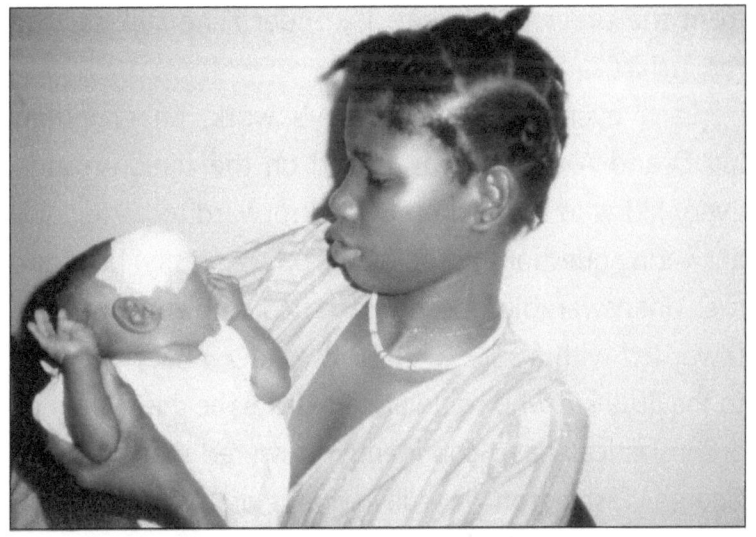

The mother of the child with bi-lateral cataracts

And John, then a four-year-old? I can still see him sitting on his mother's lap...not smiling. His infected, swollen left eye told the story of the infection, of medicine man voodoo, of being patched with no medication for two weeks. The greenhouse effect of covering an infection spells trouble: endophthalmitis. By the time his mother found the eye clinic, only the infection could be treated. The eye was lost. John was strong and stoic as a Marine and only cried a little when given a shot in his backsides. After Dr. Bryan completed the iridectomy and removed as much gunk from his eye as possible, I carried his limp wasted body to the recovery room and laid him on his right side in case he vomited. The bed was still warm from the previous patient. I wonder if he still has the red T-shirt.

Each evening, after the day's work, an enlightening Q and A session was staged on the clinic veranda. Every kid who showed up looked forward to asking and answering questions posed by the other (mostly) boys and me. Unanswerable questions and correct answers were rewarded with a stick of gum. I wonder what happened to the little kid who could already taste the gum when he enthusiastically and confidently answered that President George Washington was still in charge of the White House.

Are all these kids still alive? I wonder.

Each Sunday morning we joined throngs of sweaty African bodies as we leveraged our equally sweaty bodies against the straight backs of the overflowing pews in the Brown Memorial Chapel. Our hearts swelled as we listened to the loud wide open-mouthed singing, foot stompin' gospel songs, thunderous prayers, all tied together by a sermon that went far beyond its message. One morning the preacher spoke of a ship full of passengers tossing and heaving in the turbulent waters (uh-hun). All were dumbstruck with fear (Ooooh Lord), clutching to something for dear life, save one, a young boy who held his footing, smiling, having a marvelous time (Halleluiah). When one asked how he could be so calm and happy midst danger, he replied, "My Father's the captain" (Oooh yes, Lord, Amen).

Unshakable faith is their armor against adversity. They put their total faith in their Captain, their Papa God. Can we do any less?

"Now we are entering the rainy season and many people have no shelter, so the humanitarian situation is very acute. There are about 150,000 displaced persons in Freetown alone, with only about 30,000 of them in government camps. An epidemic of measles has caused alarm. Many children have died of measles over the past four months. Sierra Leone government and negotiators reached agreement on Thursday to allow humanitarian aid to reach starving civilians in the provinces."
Sierra Leone News, June 1999

Do we dare be optimistic?

I recall a slogan emblazoned on a moving death trap, a garishly painted bus, its bald tires bowing out under its load: HE WHO IS DOWN NEED NOT FEAR THE FALL.

Sounds like something to keep in mind when my faith gets shaky and I can't sleep.

An Easter Morning in Sierra Leone

Darkness still held on to the day when I awoke; anticipation replaced sleepiness as I listened to the beautiful rich voices wafting through our screened bedroom windows. I guessed the early risers had to be gathered within our compound since they nearly drowned out the 5:00 a.m. dissonant sounds of the Muslims' call to prayer.

As I slipped from beneath our shared mosquito netting, making sure I didn't awaken my tired husband, I noticed that two roaches had spent an over-night on top of our netting.

Pulling on yesterday's (and the day before) clothes, I quietly made my way out the clinic's upstairs living quarters, down the side stairs, hanging on to the railing to avoid any sleeping stray dogs, to the central open area of the compound.

I was not the first to arrive. I was the only white person to arrive.

Thirty or more dark shadows congregated on tired chairs, circling a bonfire blazing from the insides of an old truck tire (undoubtedly stolen), belching black acrid smoke, an anecdote to bloodthirsty mosquitoes. Voices so rich in harmony, with no need for accompaniment, rose to meet the morning. The old familiar hymn never questioned more poignantly!

"Were you there when they crucified my Lord?"

Continuing with the Easter story, we quietly and solemnly made our way to the tomb of Jesus, enhanced by cement blocks "borrowed" from a nearby construction site and a large, pummeled piece of tin, a stand-in for the rock to be rolled away.

The two Marys, with a Creole beat, wailed in question, "Where is our Jesus? Where is our Jesus?"

Jesus, shrouded in white, stood omnipotent above his disciples, one dressed in a missionary donation, a tattered plaid robe, another in faded jean cutoffs, laceless tennis shoes, and one argyle sock. There was no snickering... only reverence. I could feel the reverence. I could feel the closeness to God.

As the sun rose over the squalor of Kissy, bringing with it staggering humidity and heat, two young Africans stood before the group and gave testimony to their faith.

Energized voices, booming drums (large buckets with leather stretched across), and colorful tambourines carried the service to a dramatic (and loud—very loud) victory!

"Onward Christian Soldiers…"

With a beat that rocked my heart.

And so it was on Easter morning outside Kissy Eye Clinic, Sierra Leone, West Africa.

The Way It Was and Still Is
Ghana, West Africa

After fifteen hours wedged in an airplane seat and forty-eight hours without sleeping horizontally, you really **do** start looking like your passport photo. As my exhausted husband's head bobbed on his chest, and his body twitched in restless dozing, I sat, numb, in row 32D, and wondered if anybody would be impressed to know that he'd completed thirty-one eye surgeries, just the day before, in a Ghana, West African clinic, or that it is my birthday. Probably not.

In my sleep-deprived reverie, I thought of James and tried to imagine how it would feel to suffer a dense, rubbery mass the size of an orange wedged between my eyeball and the inside of my left lower eyelid. Seventeen-year-old James knew. This reed-thin, stoic Ghana youth, his dark eyes reflecting exhaustion, walked ten miles to the Ghanaian eye clinic, hoping the American doctor could remove his fast growing tumor…

"Are you out of Africa?" inquired the twenty-something window seat passenger, obviously pleased with her choice of words.

Not exactly a long-shot guess, considering that a couple of books on the subject bulged out of the seat pocket in front of me. When I explained that we were returning from our thirteenth trip to Africa, where my now dozing, head-bobbing husband, an ophthalmic surgeon, had completed over two hundred fifty eye surgeries in less than two weeks, she followed up with the usual bullet-type questioning: people, politics, disease, accommodations, and safety.

Sensing my lagging enthusiasm, she quickly injected, "How can you, in just one long plane ride, shift from your normal life to living with such poverty?"

"Attitude is probably the short answer," I replied.

I could tell she wanted to hear more details, but I was tired. Rudely, I laid my head back, closed my eyes, and mused. Maybe it's a story that began in conservative, small-town Iowa, pre-and post-World War II…a town where everybody knew everybody and everybody helped everybody. Maybe.

"As I walk through the villages, en route to the clinic each morning, I smile at the mamas washing their children in big

tubs. I remember my youthful Saturday night tub baths in the kitchen warmed by a coal burning cook-stove. I stand and watch them scrubbing their clothes in the streams, kids racing around the shacks, kicking homemade balls of tightly woven yarn or tin cans that some "whitey" threw out, neighbors sharing gossip as they shuck palm nuts. Why do I feel like I'm back in the 1940s rural Iowa? Maybe it's the unstructured lives of the kids. Maybe it's the heat and humidity."
                              Journal

Altoona, Iowa, (population 800) sat quietly in the middle of the state, surrounded by proud fields of corn, alfalfa, beans, productive milk cows, Iowa State Fair prize-winning hogs, and over a hundred families who showed up for every basketball and football game. Though Des Moines, the state's capital, carried on its important business only twelve miles west on Hwy 6, to an unsophisticated kid, it seemed a different world.

Altoona's L-shaped, two-blocks-long business district was creatively called Main Street. The predictable small-town businesses stood busily on either side of the street, each paying honor and attention to the popular American Legion Hall, which swept its bigness around the corner.

Altoona's folks took care of each other in sickness and in health till death did them part. The town rallied Big

Time during WWII, collecting tin cans, newspapers, and milkweed pods. (I never quite understood their purpose) Gasoline rationing kept family cars in garages. The easily recognized censored airmail letters from local service men were shared from the Sunday pulpit, and tears were shed when a boy came up missing or gold stars shone in the windows of the grieving parents, when word came, "Died in action."

"Each morning long before the sun rises to meet the day, a hundred or more African patients, on the arms of relatives, stream in from the city streets and villages, down dusty paths, their thongs and bare feet pushing clouds of red dirt off their heels, focusing their energies on getting to the clinic. The word has spread. The tall white doctor is their hope for sight.

It took three days of walking and hitchhiking through the Africa heat, over hills and plains of three countries, but 25-year old Samuel, from Guinea, was determined not to stop. He had heard about the eye clinic and he prayed someone there could fix his cornea, pierced by a nail three days before. Thankfully, the hole was stitched, antibiotics administered, and later a cataract removed and a lens implanted. I asked one of the staff about the inner strength of his people and was told they have few expectations in life and during times of pain, they just pray their way through it.

A cockroach rushed out from under the operating table to greet me this morning. I nailed him with a hard right foot."

Journal

Altoona had two churches. A Methodist church and a Christian Church of Christ. Only death kept anybody from leaving their unlocked houses and planting their Sunday shoes in one or the other. I was not inside the Methodist church until I was a teenager and sneaked in with a friend. Mom figured anybody who sprinkled their new babies must be hiding something. All members of the Christian Church had one thing in common; they had been dunked. Considering the baptismal font was the biggest body of water in Altoona, unless you counted the winter skating pond, you can understand the drama of dunking.

On the anticipated Sunday night, the soon-to-be-saved souls, dressed in assigned whites, nervous to the point of throwing up, collected in an anteroom. Clutching a white dish towel folded in fourths (ironed, of course), and with hearts pounding, each stepped blindly into the unfamiliar recesses of the chest-high tank of cold water and sloshed toward the minister. He stood, Bible in hand, braced for the event. To a twelve-year-old who had known water no deeper than a Saturday night bath in a galvanized tub, I knew this was it. I was **not** going to see my next meal.

Drowning would be listed as the cause of death in the next week's Altoona Herald.

The minister placed the cloth over my nose and mouth, and in loud Sermon-on-the-Mount tones, proclaimed, "I baptize thee in the name of the Father," (full body dunk) "the Son," (dunk) "and the Holy Ghost. Amen" (a **long** dunk); he wanted to make sure it "took".

"The young African waded hesitantly into the quiet water, tangled at the banks with undergrowth, murky from decades of abuse. He wore a frayed, terry cloth robe, once white, undoubtedly a castoff from a missionary box. The robed preacher waited in the waist-high water, his worn Bible open. He reached out his right hand to receive the youth. The baptism ceremony was about to begin. As I stood with 17-year-old Macauley's family and friends of that West African Easter Sunday morning, I smiled at the similarity of this ritual to my own baptism."

Journal

In our home, a good hot meal was a Band-Aid for most ailments, physical or emotional. A clean plate was the highest complement one could pay the cook. Armed with repeated directions for not spilling or stopping en route to talk to anybody, I hauled Thanksgiving and Christmas dinners, pies, and casseroles to two of Altoona's eccentric characters we often whispered about: Ruben Walters, a crippled bachelor who lived across the tracks, and Ell Engle, Altoona's witch in residence. Ell was always dressed in black, thin as a zipper, white hair sneaking out of a black turban; she chewed cotton with toothless gums and sat at the window of her sagging brown two-story house just two doors down from us. She liked my brother and counted on him to provide male cats, as needed, for capturing mice. Reward: 50 cents.

"As I walk through the villages to the clinic each day in Ghana or Sierra Leone, I'm greeted with friendly everyday sameness of the people's lives…of mothers who are the backbone of African life, bending over tubs or streams… cooking over an open fire pit…I see kids who are everybody's kids chasing their mangy, underfed dogs and cats, laughing, shouting, their chests bare, their feet calloused. Everybody helps everybody. Relatives lend steady hands to blind relatives making their way to the clinic; children help elderly parents and younger siblings. I see hardship. But they have what we've taken away from our generations of government-dependent families…the inner spirit to survive, to take charge of their lives, to share what they have, to value education, to not blame anybody for any misfortune, to love and to keep an unshakeable faith in God."

Journal

As I flex life back into my cramped legs, I think about my row-mate's question, of the how and why we make these trips. Actually, Africa is an annual reminder to us of what we've learned to take for granted. One of our favorite patients was an old woman, blinded with cataracts, who, the day after surgery, joyously swept around the examining room exclaiming, "I **can see**!"

Well, the Africans help us to see. Just as growing up in a small town in rural America, where interdependence, compassion, and hard work were a way of life, the Africans have given us a renewed vision of service to people.

For sure, we don't want to give up our garage door openers, indoor plumbing, instant **hot** water, or a telephone that works, but most of our possessions own us.

So are our lives planned before we're born? Were we born in small Midwestern towns to prepare our hearts and minds for work in Africa? It's tough to look back at the past and use it to explain the way life turns out. Besides, purpose and meaning of life are nearly impossible to wonder about in a muddled, travel-weary head.

As I collect myself for landing, my thoughts turn back to James, the young man with the tumor. I recall how he patiently waited until the end of the day. I see him mounting the operating table, full of optimism, situating himself, arms and hands hugging his sides. I see Dr. Bryan at the sink, scrubbing his hands, pulling on sterile gloves, sitting down at the side of James' head, gently probing, pulling, looking, thinking, then revisiting the eye under the microscope, sitting back, arms folded across his chest, his sad brown eyes peering above his sterile mask. I knew, even then, that James' tumor was more invasive than could be handled that day in the clinic.

We knew and were very sad.

Although we are often praised, stateside, for our humanitarian efforts, the truth is, it's a selfish act, really. A personal cleansing. For we look forward to shedding all the trappings advertised to ensure happiness, and once again, returning to sameness, or "the way it was"…a very long time ago.

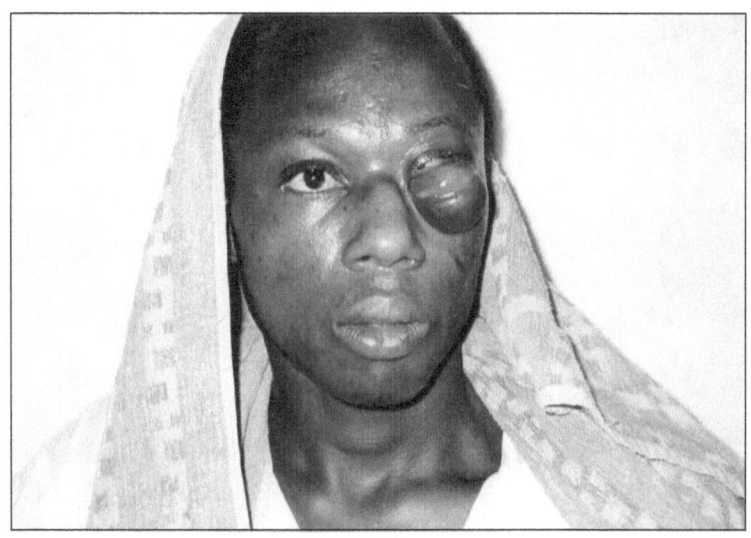

James

Ghana, West Africa
1995

The Diary of a Wife/Circulating Nurse

January 12, 1995

Yakima (Wa) airport is socked in with fog. We will be driving to Seattle.

January 13

Dare I mention it's Friday the thirteenth? We are on Alaska Air; it's 1:05 and lunch is over. We left Seattle an hour late because of weather in San Francisco, causing delays. Our Lufthansa flight is scheduled to leave at 2:35, so our concern is: WILL OUR SUPPLIES GET OFF ALASKA AND ON LUFTHANSA? The stewardess wanted us to feel confident with the fact that everything has been delayed so there probably won't be a problem. "Probably" causes us stress.

I don't know what God had to do with this, but one thing is sure. We did NOT make the flight to Ghana on Friday the thirteenth. We circled San Francisco airport for at least thirty minutes, landing, finally at 2:10. Jesse Owens would have been proud at the speed of our sprint to the check-in gate.

> WE WERE TURNED AWAY
> THEY GAVE AWAY OUR SEATS
> THERE WERE NO AVAILABLE SEATS

So began our nightmare. We stood at Lufthansa ticketing, trying, begging, to be rebooked on another airline, but because we had "bargain" tickets, Lufthansa would NOT sign off on another airline. Something to do with money. I checked with British Air who offered that they could book us right then, for $2100 ONE WAY...ONE PERSON. We declined after hearing the $2100 part. I checked with KLM via Northwest. Same response.

So after three hours of haggling, near tears, phone calls back to our travel agent in Yakima, Washington, and to Bob Ainsworth, our U.S. connection to Ghana, of explaining our mission, of how the patients will be lined up in Ghana, waiting for us, it all came down to one simple fact.

LUFTHANSA HAD GIVEN OUR CONFIRMED SEATS AWAY. Alaska lied. They had NOT bothered contacting

Lufthansa to tell them we were coming in late, but coming. The final blow came when we found out that the flight, which was supposed to leave at 2:30, did NOT leave until 3:15. We also found out that the plane WAITED for a United passenger who was late. United had called in.

So now where do we stand? Hal is ready to bag the mission, but Henry, his ophthalmic technician, and I outvoted him.

Lufthansa rescheduled us for the same flight leaving Tuesday. As the agent was checking into this, she said, "We can get you to Frankfort but the plane is booked to Accra, your destination." Then she took one look at our stricken faces and said, "We'll get you on."

Thank goodness for relatives nearby. They came, they fed us, bed us, and hauled us back to the airport on Tuesday.

January 17

As the death toll rises to 700 in Osaki/Kobe, Japan, following a twenty-second earthquake, we stood in front of the Lufthansa check-in. Again. They continued to apologize. As an apology, we didn't have to pay excess baggage on Box 7 or Henry's bag. The ticket lady further explained that the reason they waited for the United passenger last Friday was because he/she had a special "co-chair" ticket. Whatever that is.

January 19

The 19th, hopefully, since I wrote it seventeen times in the surgery logbook today. We had an hour to enjoy and walk the perimeter of Lagos, Nigeria, airport for one HOT foul-smelling hour before collecting ourselves for the last leg to Accra. We arrived on time. George, our faithful administrator, did not. After a twenty-five minute wait, we started thinking about alternatives. We had just wheeled our seven boxes to the checkout conveyor belt, handed in our passports for perusal; we knew we were in for an impossible hassle when George flew in. We discovered the office of ministry has new rules about immigrants bearing boxes but customs is not quite clear on them; they just make them up as they feel like it. We KNEW we would have been there till tomorrow morning if George had not shown up and out-talked them.

Onward to the Sunyani, clinic #1, where in record time we unpacked, shelved our supplies (the boxes became shelves), moved into the O.R., and were on our way to making up for lost time. Seventeen folks are seeing better tonight.

January 20

It's the middle of the afternoon and the electricity is down and has been for an hour. I'm sitting here in the O.R., Hal's asleep on table #2, and Henry was on the bed in the "lounge," until the jury-rigged generator woke him up. It caused the lights to flicker and even stay on for a few minutes. A patient is resting on table #1; Dr. Bryan made the initial incision BEFORE the lights went out so he put in a few temporary stitches by flashlight to hold until the electricity comes back on.

January 21

WE DID NOT GET TO BED THIS MORNING UNTIL 3:10 A.M.
TWENTY-SEVEN SURGERIES

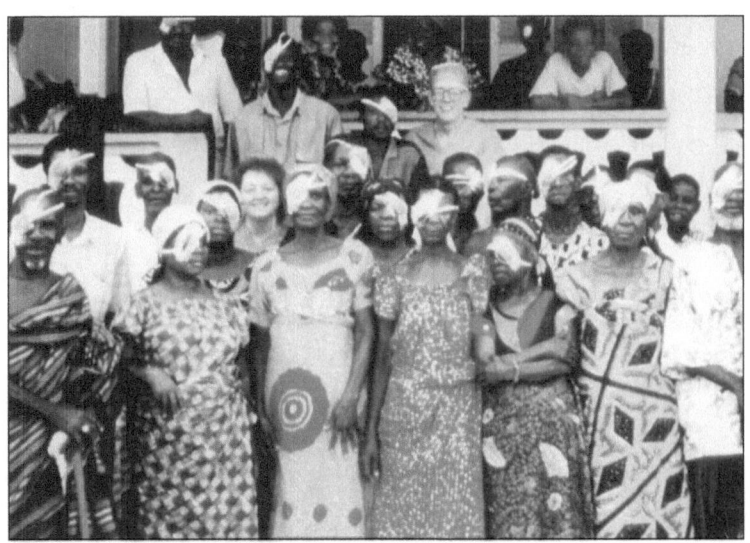

The day after surgery in Ghana

Even at that late/early hour we had hoped to have a hot shower, but no hot water, in fact no water. Found out at breakfast that it had been turned off. So, no shower. Oh, well, we'll blend in with the patients and our driver.

(If only he wouldn't rest his arm on the open windowsill as he drives us back to our room each night). We didn't wake up till 6:25 so didn't have time anyway.

So now it's 4:00:

+A patient had to be sent back because the wrong eye was blocked (anesthetized).

+The ladies of the guild came bearing food: vegetables, bread; they sang a hymn and offered a prayer during our lunch.

+The air conditioning men arrived; can't tell any difference. A lizard fell out of the A/C; I sent him on to eternity with my shoe.

+Our sleep tally:

> Wednesday night...4 hours
> Thursday night...4½ hours
> Friday night...3¼ hours

And now we are in deep do-do. Dr. Bryan's last case: 2:30 a.m. He lost vitreous, therefore an ACL lens was needed. No appropriate ACL available. Lack of sleep... lack of concentration. My mind is mush and I'm not even operating! The most memorable case today was a small boy who had a stick removed from his cornea, impressive to see the stick rise out of the pus.

Thirty-two surgeries has to be a record

January 22, Sunday

It's 9:05 and Hal is into a "combined" (cataract and glaucoma surgery) and is not happy.

First: Evelyn was late blocking a patient then did an improper lid block so we had to wait while another was blocked, THEN we discovered it was a "combined." NOT a GOOD START. We should have just gone to church.

Today we handed out T-shirts for the photo shoot; we are always short, no matter how many we haul over. We held back a special tee for Isaac; he only speaks Twi, the local language. No way could he understand my American English. Margaret, the scrub nurse, brought him to our attention. He and his two sisters are a family unit; his parents are dead. One sister is blind. Isaac, twelve years old, too, became blind. He found out about the clinic, came with a friend, and sat all day waiting for the doctor. The staff had seen him sitting, but thought he was a schoolboy just hanging around the clinic. When all the patients had been seen and he was still waiting, one of the staff asked him, "What do you want?" He said, "I am blind."

An exam revealed bilateral cataracts. Isaac was operated...it was successful; however, he will have to wear glasses that are a minus 10; since none with this correction are available here, we will send them to the clinic from the U.S.

But the most poignant moment: I wanted to get a photo of him in the T-shirt after the operation; the American in me asked him to smile. Nothing. His sister asked him. He physically could NOT smile. He exerted a big attempt to make a laugh come from his throat as in a laugh, but no smile. In human hardship ratings, he scores a solid ten. No parents, one blind sister, one sister who is trying to keep them all alive and together.

So, it's a wrap for this clinic, onward to ACCRA, the capital.

January 23

But not without adventure did we make it to Accra. We packed up and squeezed everything into George's car for a long, bumpy, hot, crowed ride to Accra. Henry took up half the back seat while Margaret, the surgical nurse, and I shared the other half.

Between Sunyani and Kumasi (the second and third clinics), George's car blew a water hose. Not to worry. A "fitter" (mechanic) showed up with a machete. He took hold of the 180-degree decayed hose, loosened the screws with an unidentifiable tool, took off the ring which secured the hose, and THEN, armed with his machete, slashed off the torn section, which fortunately was near the end, and voila...reestablished the hose to its rightful place and stretched it to its appropriate length. Sort of. Cost to him: a set of burned hands. By this time, a crowd of dozens had collected, a no-toothed skeletal man cheering on the process. Reward: the only thing we could think of: CDs to the fitter and cheerleader. Now what, I ask myself, are they going to do with the CDs, since I'm probably accurate in saying their shacks have no electricity. They'll sell them.

Onward to Accra.

January 24

Good grief. We arrived here about 9:00 last night, set up the shelving, installed the supplies, ate some stew and then to bed. BUT, we had just savored a few minutes of clean sheets in a horizontal position, under a fan, when the entire bed fell apart! The headboard and sides fell off their hinges and down we bounced. Not to worry. The mattress served its purpose on the floor. Interesting shower set up; if we want hot water we must remember to flip the right switch one hour before; therefore, a cold shower for me this morning. The fact we have to climb into a very high bathtub, stoop over because the handheld shower's hose does not reach is a small price to pay for a shower. No shower curtain, but what the…

We had a bit of a ragged start this morning. One scope doesn't work well so we put the two beds side by side with the working scope in between. Everybody has to get his/her assignment defined. Even at that, Hal managed twenty surgeries.

I walked a couple of miles this morning in the red dust of Ghana; my collection of observations includes: the Accra patients are much fatter. They don't walk as much and are better fed. The patients who are businessmen wear sox during surgery. The traders and farmers do not. Dr. Bellman (the permanent ophthalmologist from the U.S.) has "westernized" this clinic. It's much cleaner and considerably more orderly.

January 26

Where did Tuesday and Wednesday go? A blur of patients passes before my eyes. It's wonderful being able to live and operate in the same building. Hal went on the morning walk with me, but in order to do so had to wake up the night watchman to get OUT of the gate. There were at least ten folks waiting outside the gate. One of the patients complained about having to stand. Interesting, the more educated, the more complaints. The country folks just hold it in.

Most interesting case yesterday: A Tuesday post-op came back complaining of overnight pain. The tape and the shield were removed AND the underside of the shield was COVERED with red and black ants! YUK!

January 27

There were too many extraneous people in the O.R. today. It was decided yesterday that Dr. Darko, a Ghanaian ophthalmologist, should do a cataract. Dr. Bryan was into his third case when the furniture movers came in. The operating table had to be rearranged so another table could be brought into the O.R. A microscope was hauled in from the hall along with the small table with recycled gloves, gowns, etc., which required a version of sterilization to be used; the instruments had to be carried from a cabinet and sterilized.

Now Dr. Darko was ready for his patient.

Forty-five minutes later, he still was not ready to insert the lens. The microscope light went out. Henry (Dr. Bryan's technician) was rushed to the scene with two new bulbs. Neither worked. Decision: Haul Hal's finished case off the bed, push bed one to bed three slot, slide bed three with patient to slot one. Dr. Darko sat down and proceeded. He had no luck inserting the lens. Dr. Bryan took over. All movers returned to the scene to remove previous evidence. Dr. Darko went back to the observation scope and watched Dr. Bryan perform his magic.

January 29

Dr. Bryan is ready to lay down the knife on patient #200. It is 10:20 a.m.

Dr. Bryan made eighteen patients happy today, however, because of our plane schedule tonight, he had to leave a "combined" patient in the waiting room and that lady was NOT happy. Nor would I be if I'd been sitting there since 6:00 a.m.

So with Henry and George, we left the clinic one more time.

It will soon be time to reenter everyday life, an emotional transition. Hal will go back to work tomorrow. I will go back to work tomorrow. And for several weeks, we will remember; we will remember the patients whose sight was restored…we will remember the patients whose sight will never be restored…and we will look forward to next year when once again we will pack the apple boxes with four hundred to five hundred pounds of supplies and once again head to Africa.

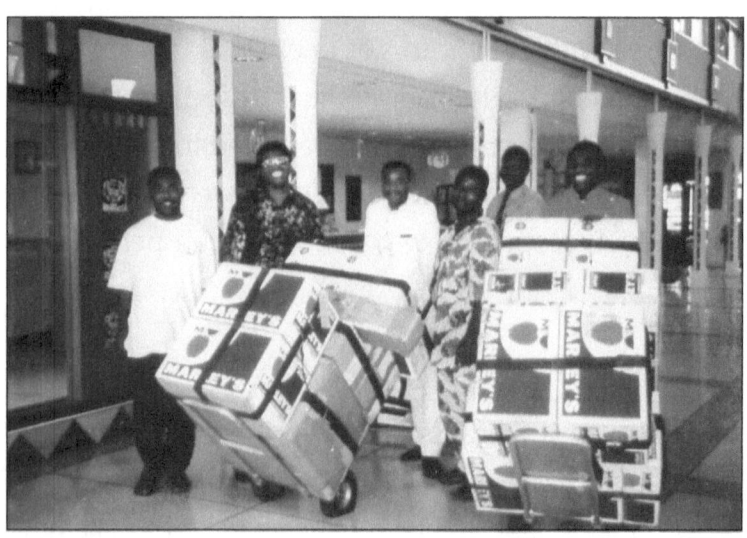

500 pounds of supplies

Haiti

As I sit hunched in front of my computer, remembering our 1985 medical eye mission in Port-au-Prince and Jacmel, I have one eye on the television showing the devastation of this island country as it recovers from a hurricane in 2010 and then flooding in 2011. I hear of the millions and millions of U.S. dollars that have flooded in there and wonder where and how it has improved the lives of Haiti's people. I see a hillside of tents, a sea of undernourished kids, defenseless against disease. I see the hopeless eyes of adults, struggling. I see health teams working day and night treating patients racked with cholera.

Haiti. Who has the answers? Where is the leadership?

Conditions were only slightly better in 1985. We saw a nation where the forests had long been felled, indiscriminately, in the name of survival, leaving unprotected land

and its crops being carried away by the heavy rains…the mountains stripped bare.

It was for the two weeks, in February 1985, that we boxed up ophthalmic supplies and left the Northwest winter to work in the clinics of Port-au-Prince and the sleepy southern coastal town of Jacmel as volunteers of Eye-Care-Haiti, a nonprofit organization.

Port-au-Prince and Jacmel
1985

> "To know one soul breathed easier
> because you lived,
> This is to have succeeded."
> Ralph Waldo Emerson

Dr. Goose is that one soul we will remember.

The calypso band was waiting for us at the Port-au-Prince airport on a warm February day. Did I say warm? The heat and humidity were staggering. Checking 500 pounds of boxed supplies through customs is never easy; curiosity is the culprit.

What are these little things?

They are put in people's eyes.

No, not possible. And this machine? A television?

No, it measures the length of eyes.

Show me.

Only when our driver came to our rescue were we excused…without the box of medicines, which they wanted to "check out". Our driver promised they would be delivered to the clinic.

For starters, the clinic was housed inside a school, a school started and administered by Sister Joan, an Episcopal nun and founding mother of L'Ecole de Vincent, a school she started under a tree with one handicapped child who needed help. Its size was the only remnant of its past haughty grandeur as a colonial mansion. The ballrooms were now a pediatric clinic, a small surgical suite, smaller classrooms, workshops operated by deaf men who made and repaired "lifts" and "legs", two dining rooms, a courtyard, and a swimming pool that looked unused and unmaintained. An eight-foot iron fence kept the kids in and the street traffic out.

All that aside, we loved the music from the still-grand entry hall that brought us awake each morning. Beautiful classical violin or piano music. We wondered, the first morning, how that could be since most of the children were blind or nearly so. We soon found out the handicap made little difference.

We met Ramel the first morning. He had no vision in one eye and only minimal sight in the other. He was an accomplished violinist, could hear a piece of music and play it. He was looking forward to an audition, which if acceptable, gave him a chance to enter Julliard. Sherry, a volunteer, tutored him for his orals. He typed his notes in Braille.

We listened in awe as Yolette played her violin; she came, often, to our room and shared that she would soon be playing a concert at Trinity Church. She also added, sadly, that she was sometimes scared and kids shunned her, undoubtedly jealous of her musical skills and the show of attention the sisters gave to her. Yolette was blind in one eye due to an injury and could only identify large shapes with the other.

Stephanie, a vamp in motion, painted lips, loopy earrings, and colorful clothes, bad skin and breath. One of many young girls taken off the streets, she had no papers so she would have been thrown in jail had it not been for St. Vincent. She informed me that I had taken a group picture that did **not** include her. She wanted **her** picture taken. She dragged a chair over, stretched a street pose, and looked right at the camera. Still in her pose, she candidly added that she had a baby boy, Jimmy, at thirteen, who lived with the father in Canada.

Many of the kids who went home for summer and Christmas vacation very often came back with bad sores, scabies, boils, malnutrition, and high fevers. Many of the blind kids were taken to the streets by their parents or older brothers and sisters, hoping to collect sympathy money.

It always takes a lot of effort to get surgery up and running in a Third World setting. The local ophthalmologist, Dr. Frederick, shared that he only operated on ten to fifteen cataracts per year at fifty dollars per surgery. It became evident the first day that Dr. Bryan's volunteer operating hands were not essential here. All was not lost, however. He assisted Dr. Frederick and a resident from Georgetown, offering key suggestions and techniques to both.

Dr. Monsanto, our host, collected us (and our supplies) for the trip to Jacmel; we left midst frantic preparations for Fat Tuesday (Mardi Gras). Little did we know what a **big** deal it really is in Haiti. The early Mardi Gras celebrants made the ride through town slow and tedious, **and** hot. It rained hard going over the mountains and caused us to miss a fantastic panoramic view; however, by the time we dipped down into much quieter, sleepy Jacmel, clear skies, beautiful green hillsides, and the Caribbean Sea welcomed us. We drove directly to the clinic and were introduced to "our house," small but colorful, and handily attached to the clinic. Dr. Monsanto waited for us to unpack before heading with us on a tour, ending at

Pension Craft to set the pattern for our eating: breakfast and a Pension lunch delivered to the clinic by our maid, Isani, and dinner at the Pension.

Hal ate goat for lunch. (Scary) I opted for the safe chicken.

The Pension was run by the iron hand of Adeline; she hands out free bread from 5:00 to 7:00 a.m. If there was any disorder among the beggars, no handouts for two days!

The balcony of the Pension was definitely the place to be. We watched the parade, smiling at a couple of kids covered in blue body paint, straddling a burro, jockeying for position; hordes and mobs of people filled the streets; tempers flared, arms and fists flailed as the sea of people pushed on.

Dr. Monsanto insisted that we continue spending our first night in Jacmel in celebration of Mardi Gras. Totally out of festive costume, we joined him and hundreds of others at a dance hall for an evening of high-octane dancing and "toasting"! Colorful costumes and handsome Haitians. By the end of the evening, no one even noticed that we were not in costume.

An interesting man, Dr. Mansanto. He trains assistants and residents, spending considerable time running back and forth between Jacmel and Port-au-Prince. He doesn't teach his assistants English because "den he leef the country." He believes that Haitian doctors should be trained in Haiti to know the Haitian problems, visit for three months in the U.S., go to meetings, work in labs, and then come back to Haiti and use what is applicable in Haiti. If they train in the U.S. and then come back to Haiti, they are frustrated with all the shortcomings of medicine in Haiti and therefore don't want to stay. The visiting physicians provide the same kind of teaching they would get in the U.S. without going there.

And **that** was what he wanted most from Dr. Bryan: teaching.

This concept was further confirmed when we talked to a wife of an osteopathic doctor from Philadelphia. Before leaving the U.S., she said she heard a news broadcast on TV featuring a health team loaded with supplies en route to Haiti; they reported that there was only one ophthalmologist in Haiti, whereas there were, we discovered upon arrival, at least fifteen in Port-au-Prince and thirteen physicians-in-training to be ophthalmologists.

What Haiti needed (and undoubtedly still needs) were more **trained** ophthalmologists, not more ophthalmologists.

We met Franz Lerge, a most handsome young man who resembled Barbarina on the old *Welcome Back Kotter* TV show. Franz, a resident in ophthalmology and an exceptional young man, spoke five languages, and lived in Port-au-Prince where his seventy-five-year-old father was also an ophthalmologist. He came to observe Dr. Bryan operate and to learn how to run the keratometer with me as the patient; he, too, thought Dr. Bryan's mission should be to teach Haitian resident ophthalmologists. (When we returned to Ecole de Vincent in Port-au-Prince en route back to the states, Franz sat down at the piano and played magnificent Chopin. We decided there was no end to this young man's talents.)

"Isani (our cook) wanted me to walk home with her to see her house. Very neat: two rooms, aqua walls, one bed, three wooden painted armed lawn chairs, small coffee table with artificial flowers in a chipped vase, a small three-legged cabinet for dishes and a collage of family pictures on the wall. In the second room, there were two beds, one bed leg residing on a concrete block to make it level, one box with a battered suitcase on it, two clotheslines with a few items of clothing, a hanging bag full of rags and underwear, three buckets of water, one briefcase full of notebooks, and an elementary textbook with its back cover missing. She pulled out pictures from the middle pages: two of Jesus and one of her at school with a friend. She wanted a photo of her at various stations 'round the house...by the door, on the porch, with flowers, slinking by the door; after each, I attempted an exit with an *au revoir, but she came back with 'no no' and then wiggled into another pose."*

Journal

With Marcel as my translator, we went to St. Michaels and visited with Sister Jane, who shared a tour with me. I witnessed a little three-year-old girl die literally before my eyes. Her young mother pulled back her covers then covered her own eyes. Sister Jane took her hand, led her out, but didn't return to the child. Later I talked to an English-speaking medic who knew the child, knew she had an intestinal disorder that, if caught soon enough, with the right antibiotics, could have been cured.

A visit to the Sisters of Charity revealed more sadness. The small children, their brown eyes looking out between the slats in their cribs, were hauntingly beautiful in their sickness. One youngster, less than a year old, was sleeping in a T-shirt emblazoned with "I LOVE MOMMY," with a Ritz cracker waiting on her shoulder. Since the Haitian women don't breastfeed, the kids have to "gum" their food early. These are the kids of the very very poor. Another room housed the older children, who were seated behind a long table with absolutely nothing in front of them to look at or do or eat. Furthermore, I could see nothing anywhere in the room for them to do. Their hair was various shades of dull and lifeless brown, which smacked of malnutrition.

One of the sisters from Belgium explained they had to now keep the gate locked and parents' visitation limited to Sundays only because the parents stole them blind. One week alone, sixteen bed sheets disappeared. At Christmas time, huge boxes of toys arrived from the United States, and within two weeks all but a very few disappeared. The children, for the most part, are brought to the sisters because of malnutrition. One mother, seven months pregnant, arrived to pick up her child, undoubtedly to be used for street begging. By the end of the weekend, the child would predictably be returned in worse condition.

I read, "A man would rather let his child go hungry than milk his goat. To do so would imply that he was poor."

We watched an old lady squatting on a stool folding hospital sheets that had dried on the grass stubble. Dr. Monsanto said the oxygen from the grass bleaches the white clothes. We wondered how that was possible considering the clouds of dust and dirt **everywhere**. We even spit dust in the sink when we brushed our teeth!

We know for sure, if it were not for Franz at Dr. Bryan's elbow, it would be impossible to take any history from the patients. As mentioned before, Dr. Monsanto encouraged **no** English. He mentioned that his secretary recently pushed him for more money. Eye Care pays part of the salaries and Dr. Monsanto pays the rest to reach a total of $250 a month. As he reminded us, the better they get, the more demands they make.

Enter Dr. Goose, happily tottering around the hospital on the hill!

Dr. Goose is a legend in Haiti. A round dough-boy shape of a man, a shock of thick white hair over a round almond face, shaggy white brows hovering over twinkling small brown eyes, eighty-two-year-old Dr. Goose never married, but reportedly sired fifty-two children. Only half as many as his father, according to the wags. He lived where he worked; in fact, he often saw his patients as he lay in bed! Dr. Goose had cataracts. He knew he had cataracts. Considering he saw 20/400, he was encouraged to have them removed but, over the years, refused time and again.

When we arrived at the hospital for our first meeting, a young woman was lying on an exam table with a belly that looked nine months pregnant. Without formal greeting, Dr. Goose asked Dr. Bryan to take a look. Hal palpitated the belly and could only guess: Fibroid cyst? Cancerous tumor of the uterus? She was later sent away for an X-ray.

Hal also looked in on an emaciated young woman who had been abandoned by a stepfather who sent her from Port-au-Prince: dehydrated, vomiting, diarrhea; it was easy, however, to observe that Julie was once a very pretty young woman.

The morning of Dr. Goose's clinic exam, Franz and Dr. Bryan collected Dr. Goose and checked in on Julia.

Franz thought she probably had AIDS; we learned from Dr. Goose that she used to be a prostitute, plump and sassy and pretty until her boyfriend pimp got mad at her and kicked her in the stomach. That was the beginning of her downfall. She was now skin and bones. On a return trip, I carried along some hot oatmeal, evaporated milk, granola bar, and then fed her. She had never tasted oatmeal.

The day of Dr. Goose's surgery arrived, however, the president decided the day should be a holiday to rest up after the holidays. No surgery. Besides, though Dr. Goose came to the clinic, he hadn't totally decided to have the surgery!

Once again, the day of surgery arrived, as did Dr. Goose. **Finally**. Dr. Bryan first maneuvered Dr. Goose's inverted right eyelid lashes back to their natural site rather than sticking in his eye. Then, before Dr. Goose could change his mind, Dr. Bryan quickly continued with cataract surgery with a lens implant in his left eye.

It was textbook perfect. By 5:00, the whole town knew that Dr. Goose had received two new eyes by the American doctor. Hal thinks that Dr. Goose thinks that he, Hal, was from Washington, D.C., or New York. "I heard you were coming before you come," said Dr. Goose.

I later met a lady on the street who asked if I lived in Jacmel. In my stumbling French, I explained, "eye doctor," and she replied, "Oh oui…doc-tor Goose…cat-a-rakt. Tres bien."

On our last night in Jacmel, we once again met for dinner at the Pension Craft. By then we knew the menu by heart and vowed not to eat any more meat. We watched a wedding reception from across the room; the groom was an employee of the Pension and obviously had not chosen his bride for her dazzling smile. As he approached the wedding cake, the sweating groom was asked if f he could "cut it." "No," he said, he could not "cut it." And then everyone laughed big time. The two Americans were helped along with the explanation: in Haitian culture, "to make sex" is "to cut it."

Later, the visiting health team decided we couldn't leave Haiti before participating in a voodoo ceremony. We joined a dozen curiosity seekers in a lantern-lit backyard and collected under an open thatched-roofed enclosure, held upright by four unstable poles pounded into the water-starved soil. We were put into the mood with wild drums booming, voices chanting, young men jumping and writhing. PETRO VEVER was outlined very artistically, in corn meal, in the middle of the dirt floor, by a young man draped in black. A bottle of rum was passed around while a wild-eyed, barefooted woman, draped in various yards of color, flailed herself around, shaking hard the hands of everyone, waking up a little kid leaning against a post. We couldn't see much happening after the wild and crazy intro so left before whatever climax was planned, thereby skipping out on the two bucks per person tab. I guess we were expecting magic; maybe too many "blancos" (white folks). But what about the words PETRO VEVER? We have no idea.

Medically, Dr. Bryan was disappointed the Mardi Gras holiday interrupted the scheduled surgery; however, we were able to see the country and get involved in the lives of many of its people. We are grateful. And besides, we are blessed that Dr. Goose finally put his trust and his eyes in the hands of Dr. Bryan.

We will not forget him.

To know we've made life easier for just one, made the trip worthwhile.

Eyes on the Philippines

It's no secret to us why General McArthur announced in 1944 that he **would** return. The warm temperatures of January and February were exceeded only by the warmth of the Filipino people. So how did we happen to choose their largest island of Luzon, the province of Pangasinan, the city of Dagupan? Because of one man... Gil De Venecia, an ophthalmologist and professor at the University of Wisconsin, who grew up in Dagupan City and has taken-on the mission of providing eye care for indigent eye patients. He collects donations and services of ophthalmologists and heads over there for six weeks each year, a modest amount of time in relation to the need.

Gil often talked of the Japanese occupation. Though he lived in the province of Dagupan and witnessed many air attacks, his family had food and were relatively secure so long as they turned to the east each morning and bowed when they walked by the sentries each morning. Gil was ten years old, so he saw the war as a bit more exciting than the adults. He went on to add that the Japanese were masters of torture and would do so in order to get information out of people, especially about the whereabouts of the guerillas, who were hiding in the Baguio Hills. He remembered, too, the day an American plane was hit, the pilot parachuted out, and unfortunately, used as target practice.

Mangatarem Provincial Hospital was our destination each morning. We drove through the early morning countryside for about an hour to reach the low, cement, one-story structure with a broad veranda. The corridors and small recovery rooms were a kaleidoscope of small brown bodies, assorted cots, two to a surface, feet to heads; mats and blankets blocked off corners of people as they collected, prepared, and ate their food, and cared for their recovering relatives.

This, then, was the setting for our mission.

Doctor, Heal Thyself
The Philippines,
Pangasinan Province
1989

It's tough to fall asleep in an unoccupied house with a bayonet bracketed above your bed. Too, the bed sheets held the musty scent of the closed, unused room, opened in the middle of the night by a tired caretaker to accommodate us for our few remaining hours in the Philippines.

The next morning, over breakfast, our host, Dr. Renee Santos, an orthopedic surgeon, shared that his father, General Santos, whose memorabilia filled our bedroom and our dreams, escaped from the infamous 1941 Bataan death march to lead a pack of guerillas into the hills against the Japanese.

Dr. Santos mused, "As an eight-year-old, I looked so Japanese that I could walk by the Japanese sentries with messages and a gun in my bag!" Then, as an afterthought, he tactfully inquired if we had slept well.

We lied.

Lifting his coffee cup, he added, "All the massive, dark furniture in the house was carved by prisoners when my father was Director of Prisons."

En route to the airport later that morning, we reflected on our previous three-week eye mission outside Manila, in the province of Pangasinan. "Frankly," I sighed to my exhausted husband, "I think Dr. C. is still sore at America."

We both remembered our first serious dinner conversation with Dr. C. Her delicate jaw set, black eyes flashing, and rising to her full lovely five feet, hands on her narrow hips, she passionately lashed out, "When Japan invaded the Philippines, our home was burned and my family escaped midst bayonets and gun fire. But when the war was over, what did the United States do? They gave **more** money to Japan to rebuild than to the Philippines!"

We had no rebuttal. She expected none.

It was evident from the first day in surgery that Dr. C, a visiting Filipino ophthalmologist, saw no need for the tall, middle-aged American ophthalmologist to be at the

Mangatarem Clinic, preferring, instead, to secure the operating room and the blind patients to her skills.

Each morning, she didn't walk but rather sprinted from the car to lay claim to the better of the two operating microscopes. From her stool she didn't budge, except on the morning the scope's light bulb burned out and she insisted that Dr. Bryan leave his patient and let her use his inferior, but at least working, microscope. Fortunately, having encountered every challenging surgical, mechanical, and personnel problem during previous Third World eye missions, he had learned to negotiate faulty equipment in operating room conflicts. If anyone were keeping score in that room, they would have noted that Dr. Bryan not only found a replacement but also finished not only one, but two patients in the same amount of time that his determined team member completed one surgery.

The waiting patients knew nothing of the quiet battle over space and microscopes as they queued up, dozed in the sun, or hunkered in a squat to eat their rice and beans.

Nearly matching his weight with his years, seventy-five-year-old Solomon, bony back curved with scoliosis, face lined with wear and tear of age and hardship, head bald, eyes blinded for many years by cataracts, was led to the clinic by his wife. On cue, Dr. Bryan, a giant by comparison, carried him into the operating room.

When Solomon's taped eye patch was removed the following morning, he produced a gummy grin and demanded, "Where's my wife? I want to see my wife again."

His size-four wife, white hair coiled on top of her head, a sparkle in her brown eyes, shook Solomon by the shoulder and announced, "Hey, old man, I'm your wife. I'm standing right here in front of you!"

"No, no, no, you **can't** be my wife. You don't have any teeth and you're old." Fortunately, he wrapped his bony, arthritic arms around her frail body before she could deck him.

As with Solomon, ninety-year-old Benito, thin as a reed, light as a feather, was carried to the operating table. When his patch was removed the next morning, he was **so** happy he could see.

"Now I can see the chicks. Where are the chicks?" he asked. He continued to ogle all the women, who, on cue covered their mouths and tittered. He turned to Dr. Bryan and said, "I want to make the other eye see."

When Dr. Bryan asked why, Benito replied, "So I can see **more** chicks."

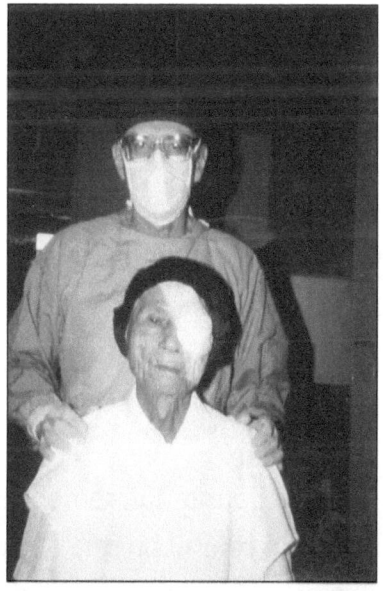

He just wanted to see the "chicks"

"Traveling to and from the clinic each day provided not only a visual overload for us, but we were a captive audience for Dr. C's coverage of World War II. 'Americans can't imagine the agony and terror of war on their homeland,' she second guessed, 'or of being forced to watch the enemy rape and loot, of going without food'. I didn't think she wanted to hear about American losses...

A bit shamelessly, I sometimes tuned her out and marveled, instead, at the skill and courage required to pedal the adult tricycles piled dangerously high with baskets, or the crazy jumble of outrageously painted, trolley-like jeepneys, all exceeding the passenger limit by at least a dozen. Horns blaring, dodging in and out of the traffic, caravans of Brahmans, ambled confidently down the narrow streets, oblivious to the roar of traffic, seemingly confident that they would NOT be sacrificed. One of the most curious sights on the ride each morning was the rice dumped on the highway to dry. What was truly amazing was that the traffic drove AROUND the rice...not through it!"

Journal

Pelagia Ramos undoubtedly remembered General MacArthur's promise to return, but the day of her cataract surgery, it didn't matter. "My body is still good, so please, Doctor," she pleaded, "fix my eye so I can see."

Removing post-operative eye patches always provides high drama. Pelagia's reaction was no exception. "Can you read the eye chart behind me?" queried Dr. Bryan. No response. He patiently stood and walked to the chart, then peering over his dark-rimmed glasses, asked again, "Can you see this chart?"

Pelagia, pepper-gray hair stretched into a tight knot on her crown, brown age spots dotting her almond face, broke into a broad chipped-tooth grin, "I can see." Then louder, "I can see, I can SEE, I CAN SEE!" Then she danced around the room hugging everybody, proclaiming to the whole clinic, "I CAN SEE!"

We will not forget eleven-year-old Samuel. It was hard not to stare at him. Born with a severe cleft lip, he endured grotesque disfigurement and a severe speech impairment. Where his mouth and upper lip should have been, only a hole resided; a red gum and a misdirected tooth filled the hole that ran to his nose. Samuel became my shadow the day he arrived with his grandmother. She was there for cataract surgery while he and the rest of his family were there for support, not an uncommon arrangement. The sterilizing setup for the surgical instruments was a kettle of boiling water on a hot plate, which claimed a spot on the floor outside the operating room and down the hall. Samuel was curious about what I was doing and followed me from the O.R. on each of my many trips as I carried instruments to and from the operating room. We carried on a one-way conversation...I talked, he listened. How much of my English bantering did he understand, I don't know, but he liked the activity to be sure. A bright red T-shirt emblazoned with a Coca-Cola logo only enhanced his devotion. That word he **did** understand.

I asked the staff about the availability of oral surgery in Manila; they readily shared that there was more than one competent surgeon. They wasted no time making an appointment to have Samuel's cleft palate and lip reconstructed, and were grateful to know that Dr. Bryan would pick up the tab. We were very excited and couldn't wait to share the news with Samuel's family, who in turn became excited and, in their own language, passed along the good news to Samuel.

At 8:00 p.m. on our last day of surgery, we prepared to pack up and to say goodbye to everyone, when one of the staff came hurriedly to me and said, "Samuel is not sure he wants to go through with the surgery."

I wasted no time asking the staff person to lead me to Samuel, his recovering grandmother and sleeping family. Down the hall, to a small, dark, windowless room strewn with mats, we wakened Samuel, brought him to the hallway, and, with sleep still covering his face, sat him knee to knee with me.

"Samuel, I understand you're thinking you won't have surgery." (Translation)

"Just think," I went on, "you'll be able to eat better."

No response.

"You'll be able to go to school and learn to read."

No response.

"You'll be able to talk, you will be such a handsome eleven-year-old."

No response.

"Samuel," I repeated, "if you will have the surgery, Dr. Bryan and I will make sure you get a new red bicycle."

Big response. His black eyes grew wide, his twisted mouth, what there was of it, twitched in anticipation of a gift so coveted!

Dr. C discovered that Dr. Bryan and I had arranged Samuel's corrective oral surgery **and** a promise of a red bicycle. As the staff circled us to say goodbye, she edged forward, looked up at Dr. Bryan, offered her hand, and said, "I heard what you are doing for Samuel. Thank you." Then, turning to leave, she glanced back over her shoulder, "And…thank you for coming."

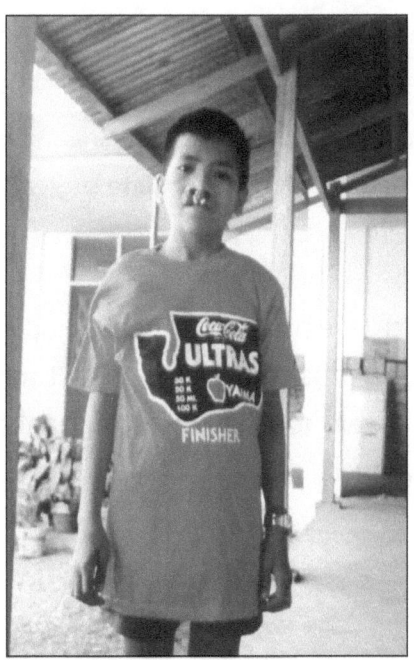

Samuel before cleft palate surgery

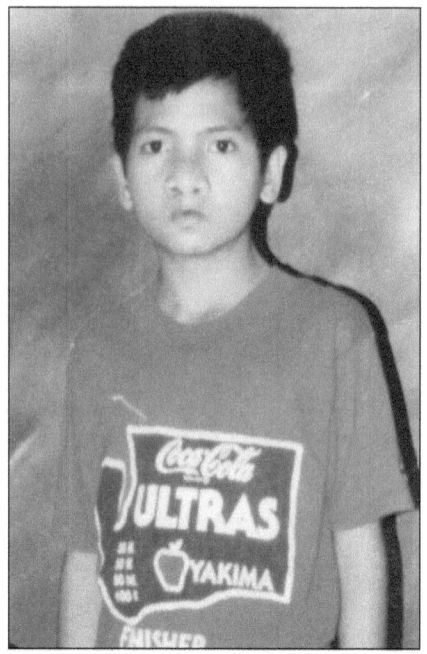

Samuel after cleft palate surgery

Postscript:

Samuel **did** have successful surgery, and he **did** get the bicycle. Not red, but blue, but he didn't mind. Samuel's father wrote a very touching note of thanks for giving a new life to Samuel.

Creatures of the Night

As we lie on our well-worn, thin mattresses, with histories of many volunteer bodies, bedsprings attempting to be noticed in our backs, heads on lumpy, musty-smelling pillows, waiting for sleep to come, we always are wary of the creatures of the night. We can hear them. They scrape their spiny legs, wispy wings, antennae, or whatever, in the corners of our bedroom, up the walls, and under our bed. Occasionally, the air-enhanced species fly over our heads.

I suck in my breath as I remember one night in the Philippines.

I was awakened by something crawling, no, not crawling, but racing, up the inside of my right thigh at a rate fast enough for me to waste no time as I yanked off the thin sheet and grabbed at the intruder.

Crunch!

I didn't know what **it** was till morning's first light when I slid out of bed and saw the mangled carcass of a two-inch cockroach. **Yikes!**

I'm lucky to be a light sleeper! I dare imagine the intruder's final destination!

Rockin' and Rollin'
Guatemala, Santo Tomas
El Salvador, La Union

It was rock-and-roll time in the operating room on the Caribbean Mercy ship! Without the music.

An enormous ship, it was, and though docked, it still rocked and rolled; the operating microscope, anchored to a plank, offering some stability, but even at that, Dr. Bryan's shoulders ached at the end of the day from leaning hard into the microscope, hands firm against the foreheads of the patients. Adhesive tape was often required to keep the patients' heads steady.

The Caribbean Mercy, formerly a Norwegian ferry, was one of several nongovernmental hospital ships throughout the world; in addition to providing health care, its volunteers also completed construction of houses and schools as well as digging wells and other agriculture projects in developing nations.

Though providing eye care served a critical need, evangelism ranked as a high priority on the Caribbean Mercy. We witnessed firsthand a discipleship training school where young adults spent nearly five months in lectures, evangelism, and working on projects with existing missionaries while demonstrating the love of God in the towns and villages.

Two objectives became clear to us. The first day taught us that surgery would not start until after morning worship, and when the quitting bell rang at 5:00, all work ceased. However, after two days of haggling, the head of the O.R. finally relented; the patients would be "blocked" before worship, and surgery would follow.

During an evening dinner conversation, one of the staff emphatically remarked, "You can get to heaven with a cleft palate or a blind eye, but you can't get there unless you know Jesus."

Our response: "What did Jesus do when he saw a lame man, a blind man, a dead man? He didn't first ask them of their beliefs."

First, He healed.

Our mission remained: treat as many blind eyes as possible. It's always the patients we remember.

* * *

Looking back, a slide show of faces of patients, events, and conflict clicks through my head.

Click: I see Juan, a cataract patient. Juan was on his back, ready for surgery, when Mike, an O.R. circulator, bent within inches of Juan's face, then, in loud accusing tones, asked if he had accepted the Lord. When the patient, sweat bubbling on his forehead, fingers twitching under the surgical sheet, said yes, Mike went on to ask how he knew.

"What do you believe?"

Juan became a fifth-grader, laid flat on the playground with the school bully on top of him. Juan kept telling Mike that he prayed, read his Bible, was a Lutheran, but Mike kept on him, his broad face, looming down, practically screaming.

"But do you know what you believe?"

It became obvious that Juan thought he had to respond with a passionate **yes**, or he'd get pulled off the table and sent home, a doomed man.

I regret not pulling Mike aside and saying, "Juan's business is with God, not with you."

* * *

Click: High drama. Guatemala's First Lady was scheduled to tour the ship on Monday and to watch cataract surgery, which was a new service added to Mercy's outreach. Her date: Monday. 11:00 a.m. The O.R. head nurse's assignment: Choose the "perfect" cataract. Translation: No apparent complications. The First Lady did not arrive until 12:10, went first to the clinic, where Henry screened patients, then to the O.R.

Trailing her was her lady-in-waiting, an interpreter, public relation person, and a (sweating) guy with a huge video camera who tried to put the camera lens next to the teaching arm of the microscope to film the surgery. It didn't work. Add Brett, the CEO of the Mercy Ship. **All** of these folks in the O.R. with us, all of us gowned, masked, and shod in sterile (sort of) booties, all the visitors trying to see **in** the microscope or over Dr. Bryan's shoulder. My claustrophobia kicked in, demanding I ease toward, then quickly through the door without, hopefully, bumping into royalty.

But she was too late to observe the original choice of patients for surgery. Dr. Bryan's final stitches closed the wound of patient number one, as her highness swept through the door. The second patient was rolled in, prepped, and made ready for surgery. Though initial incisions are small and nearly bloodless, **she had enough. That was it. She wanted to see no more.** She and her entourage tore off gowns and face masks and fled in one desperate swoop!

And a good thing.

Just as the O.R. was cleared of royalty, the insides of the patient's eye totally expulsed; blood, vitreous and capsule all spewed out like a lanced boil.

Not good P.R. Not a good clip on the evening news.

* * *

Click: A coincidence. The Holland Cruise ship docked alongside the Caribbean Mercy and tourists spilled out, eager to find souvenirs to haul home in their suitcases, never to be looked at again. The captain of the Holland came over to the Caribbean Mercy and remarked to someone,

"That ship looks familiar."

After closer observation, he discovered the Caribbean Mercy is the ship his father captained off the coast of Norway when the observing captain was a little boy. The Mercy Ship folks bought the Caribbean from a Norwegian company.

* * *

Click: Two weeks ago the O.R. supervisor dug in her heels about blocking patients **before** morning worship. BUT she relented and is glad of it. Record number of surgeries!

An efficient O.R. does not interfere with God's work...it enhances it.

She served cake.

A dead fly was stuck in the frosting

* * *

Click: Moses, a lively shadow on the ship most every day, was ten years old, but looked much younger carrying his forty-five pounds of body weight. I joined some of the staff for a short walking trip to Moses' house-to-be, a 20x20-foot structure. The footings were in, their previous shack torn down, and the cement blocks ready to be cemented together. The whole miserable grassless real estate looked like Africa with its piles of ragged timbers, metal pieces lying about, red dust over everything, wild pigs imprisoned in a fenced area just beyond the construction site. I met Mama, much older Papa, and two little girls who, when they saw us, rushed inside their temporary shack to put on new dresses, a gift from the Mercy crew. Elder son, Roberto, fourteen, works fourteen hours a day, five days a week and seven hours on Saturday in a bakery. Three dollars a day.

* * *

Click: Our first Salvadorian patient: Senovia Romero, age ninety, deaf and blind. One eye was gone and a dense cataract resided in the other. She was a problem from the get-go, wailed during the "blocks" and picked up speed from there. She flailed her head around until we had to tape it down. Every touch was a rape of her soul, till finally, she cried that she wanted to go home. Fortunately, Dr. Bryan had only made a conjunctival incision when she reached her final crescendo. Surgery halted, the wound cauterized and she bailed out of the operating room. Silly me, I held out till the end with bribes of nice hymns from the cassette player. I forgot she was deaf.

* * *

Click: Greg, an optometrist, and I walked down a rocky path and up a hill to the last gate guarding the La Union docking area, to see a family he knew from the ship. It was dusk, so though I met each family member, the growing darkness negated any clear character sketch. No electricity, no running water, and ragged burlap bags for rugs on a swept dirt floor. Papa, retired as chief administrator of the guards and dock, received no money but his family had permission to stay forever in their house on this property. Papa died of a broken heart after Son #1 was murdered in La Union two years ago. So Mama, who's lived in the shack for forty years, now shared it with her children, grandchildren, and another wife or two. She made her living cooking meals for the guards, for twenty-five cents a day. They were so gracious and hospitable, and asked us to sit a bit; chickens, dogs, cats, baby chicks ran in and out of the house like children and sat on the furniture as if they belonged there. One kid put a cloth over a chicken on a chair. The chicken settled down for the night until a dog came by, whisked the cloth off, at which point the chicken started chasing the dog in and out, round and about until the chicken tired of the game and the dog became interested in the blue bag I'd brought along.

* * *

Click: We never saw eye to eye with L. regarding prayer. She distributed slips of paper every morning, each with a patient's name, then asked us to pray for that patient. Dr. Bryan refused a slip by saying, "When I sit down in front of a patient, I pray for each one of them silently. And I don't have to worry about getting the name right since God already knows each one by name."

No rebuttal.

* * *

Click: Made a trip with Henry to the hospital in La Union; its cleanliness amazed and surprised me. We found Sirguro, a patient who had to be rescheduled because of high pressure in his eye. His pressure had dropped to 31. Good news. Saw three new babies suckling their mothers in the hall. A young woman was brought in to the emergency room, the feet and legs of her baby already birthing! Tim, the ship doctor, and a couple of residents just happened to be there. Thankfully. A breach birth. Tough but accomplished by Tim, who hadn't delivered a baby since internship!

* * *

Click: Tension on the dock! Dr. Bryan noticed that one of the nurses was not taking pressures correctly, but when he tried to show her how and why it should be taken the standard way, **all** the nurses arched their backs and held their ground. "This is how we're supposed to take it," they curtly replied (without looking at him).

Ouch!

An example of their findings: their pressure result on a patient was 36, and Henry's was 16. A **huge** difference when it comes to the health of a patient's eye!

Accepting change is tough.

* * *

Click: One more look at Moses' family's house. The roof is on and all but the last layer of floor is laid. How do the neighbors feel about this gift? Left out? I'd be envious, but according to the volunteer builders, the neighbors rejoice in their neighbors' blessings. Papa is in his seventies so it will be nice for him to have a dry home when the spring rains come and his old bones creak.

* * *

It's easy to compare working on the ship in a sterile environment versus in the clinics of Africa, Haiti, Philippines, where everything is recycled, used, and reused, but in the end, the common thread is the patient and the critical need for eye care. It's wherever we haul our five hundred pounds of supplies.

Time to go home.

And Finally…

Jabwana sat stoically as Dr. Bryan examined her newly operated eye. It was her face that held my attention; a ring snaked its way through the septum of her nose, a gold bead decorated the left flare of her nostril, and gold rings bordered the outside edges of each ear, complementing scalloped holes in her earlobes. Voodoo elephant-hair bracelets hid her weathered wrists and forearms. We learned these were to ward off evil spirits and, undoubtedly, mistakes by American doctors.

Sweat poured off her broad bare chest and breasts, which hung like empty black pockets. She was scared to death. No smiles from this lady!

"What's wrong, Jabwana? Aren't you happy?" asked Dr. Bryan. "Yesterday you could see nothing. Today you can see."

She waited, then ever so quietly replied, "I happy on inside."

On each mission, Dr. Bryan did all he could to save and improve sight, but the African, Haitian, Guatemalan, El Salvadorian, and Filipino people paid us back in full, for they filled our hearts and, as Jabwana said, they made us feel "happy on inside."

What greater gift than that?

Albert H. (Hal) and Greta Bryan are native Iowans. However, they have resided the past forty years in Yakima, Washington, where Hal practiced ophthalmology. He graduated from the University of Iowa medical school, and interned in the San Joaquin General Hospital, outside of Stockton, California, before returning to the university for a residency in ophthalmology. Greta graduated from the University of Iowa, and taught fifth grade before heading to Washington, where she directed an outreach program at the local YMCA for twenty years before retiring.

The Clinics

Though each of the clinics was created and funded under different organizations, and, in two cases, private individuals, Dr. Bryan funded our air transportation as well as his ophthalmic technician, Henry McClamrock, and scrub nurse, Bonnie Huntzinger. We are grateful to them for their service and good humor and to the many drug companies for their generosity in supplying lenses, eye drops, and disposables, i.e., needles used for injections, bandages, gloves, eye patches, drapes, gowns, etc.

+Sierra Leone, West Africa
   The Kissy Eye Clinic
   Outside of Freetown.
   Though the Methodists served as a conduit, the clinic was built by donated funds and volunteer help, directed by Dr. Lowell Gess.

+Haiti
   Eye Care Haiti
   Port-au-Prince
   Jacmel

+Ghana, West Africa
   Unite for Sight
   Accra
   Sunyani
   Cape Coast

+Kenya, East Africa
   Lighthouse for Christ
   Mombasa

+Philippines
   Dagupan City, Pangasinan Province, island of Luzon
   The success in securing donations and volunteer ophthalmologists for the clinic in the Mangatarem Provincial Hospital is due to the efforts of Gil De Venecia, M.D.

+The Caribbean Mercy Ship:
   Non-governmental worldwide hospital ships
   Guatemala: Santo Tomas
   El Salvador: La Union

Destinations

We spent two to four weeks on each mission.

1984   Sierra Leone

1985   Haiti

1986   Sierra Leone

1987   Kenya

1988   Kenya

1989   Philippines

1990   Ghana

1991	Ghana
1992	Sierra Leone
1993	Ghana
1994	Ghana
1995	Ghana
1996	Ghana
1997	Guatemala
1999	El Salvador

Definitions

CATARACT: Clouding of the lens of the eye

GLAUCOMA: Increased pressure inside the eye

"A COMBINED": Cataract and glaucoma operations at the same time

KERATOMETER: A machine that measures the curvature of the front surface of the cornea; needed to compute the power of the lens

LENS IMPLANT: Artificial lens used to replace a cataractous lens removed from the eye

ANTERIOR CHAMBER LENS: Artificial lens implanted in front of the iris (anterior to the iris)

POSTERIOR CHAMBER LENS: Artificial lens implanted behind the iris, preferably in the lens capsule

BLOCK: Injection used to produce anesthesia

VITREOUS: A clear, jelly-like material inside the posterior part of the eye, behind the lens and the iris

CONJUNCTIVA: Filmy transparent layer over the white part of the eye

SCRUB NURSE: Assists surgery by handing sterile instruments to the ophthalmologist and sometimes acting as an assistant to the doctor; always sterile

CIRCULATING NURSE: The head nurse ("boss") of the operating room (O.R.). She/he is the one who carries out the non-sterile duties in the operating room required to assist the surgeon and the scrub nurse

www.ingramcontent.com/pod-product-compliance
Lightning Source LLC
Chambersburg PA
CBHW022022170526
45157CB00003B/1321

9781460948774